T0153434

the little book of HERBALISM and natural healing

Published by OH!
20 Mortimer Street
London W1T 3JW

Disclaimer:
This book and the information contained herein are for general educational and entertainment use only. The contents are not claimed to be exhaustive, and the book is sold on the understanding that neither the publishers nor the author are thereby engaged in rendering any kind of professional services. Users are encouraged to confirm the information contained herein with other sources and review the information carefully with their appropriate, qualified service providers. Neither the publishers nor the author shall have any responsibility to any person or entity regarding any loss or damage whatsoever, direct or indirect, consequential, special or exemplary, caused or alleged to be caused, by the use or misuse of information contained in this book.

ISBN 978-1-91161-089-2

Editorial consultant: Sasha Fenton
Editorial: Victoria Godden
Project manager: Russell Porter
Design: Ben Ruocco
Production: Rachel Burgess

A CIP catalogue record for this book is available from the British Library

Printed in China

10 9 8 7 6 5 4 3 2 1

the little book of HERBALISM and natural healing

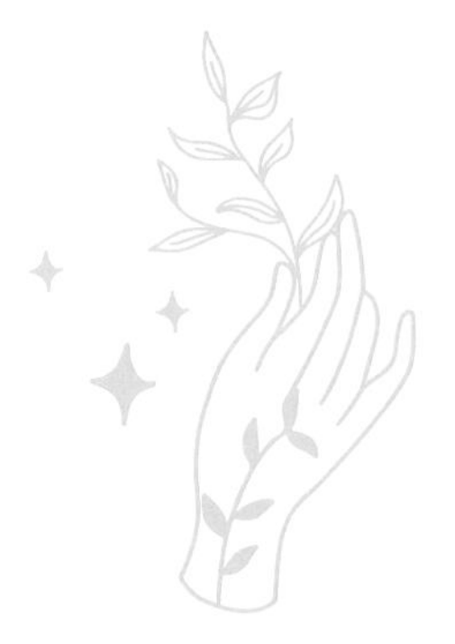

marlene houghton PhD

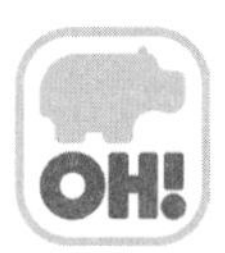

CONTENTS

INTRODUCTION

The Lord hath created medicines out of the earth and he that is wise will not abhor them.
Ecclesiasticus 38:4–5

This book is an introductory guide to the fascinating world of traditional herbalism. Herbal medicine and the use of herbs to address health issues is the oldest form of treatment known to human beings, and it is still widely used all over the world. Herbalism, also known as phytotherapy, is the therapeutic use of plants as medicine for holistic healing and healthcare.

Herbs can also be used for preventative purposes and as healthcare agents to treat common, everyday ailments. Herbal medicine is used to stimulate and strengthen the body's functions and to encourage the body to heal itself. For centuries, herbs have also been used to add spice and flavour to many kinds of food, and their use as medicine dates back to ancient history – the earliest recorded is by the Sumerians 5,000 years ago. Herbal medicine is not an allopathic discipline (a standard medical discipline), but an alternative one, though it can also be used in a complementary way, alongside mainstream medicine.

CHAPTER 1

ABOUT HERBALISM

Used in conjunction with contemporary Western medicine, herbs combine the benefits of centuries of traditional knowledge and wisdom with what is today called integrative medicine.

In the West, we now have the use of many herbs from diverse cultures; herbs from Traditional Chinese Medicine and Indian herbs from Ayurvedic medicine.

Traditional Chinese Medicine (TCM) has existed for over 4,000 years and is a medical system with its own principles that include herbal treatment. TCM assesses the life force – "qi" – a subtle, intangible, invisible energy that cannot be scientifically proven.

The Chinese believe this force flows throughout the body, and the TCM system is based on "qi" as well as the theory of yin and yang (the harmony of seemingly opposite forces).

Health and illness can be understood as having two aspects, and in a healthy body, these are in balance. If these energies are out of balance, TCM seeks to repair any deficiency with herbs, foods or acupuncture.

Ayurveda is an ancient Indian healing philosophy that assesses what are believed to be the three primary life forces of the body, or "doshas", and divides the body into three constitutional types.

Although these systems differ in their approach, the ultimate goal of both TCM and Ayurvedic medicine is to restore health to the body by restoring balance.

In Western herbalism, health is viewed as a positive state, and disease, or "dis-ease", is seen as a sign of disharmony in the body. To restore homeostasis (i.e. to take people back to good health), herbs and plants are used to increase the body's vital life force.

The overall aim of herbal medicine is to prevent disease by using herbs. When disease does occur, the objective is to enhance the body's own healing defences and to minimize the length of the illness.

These three systems, although appearing philosophically different, all use nature's plants and herbs to promote good health.

In the West, the more exotic Chinese and Indian herbs that had not been heard of years ago are now easily obtainable in health food shops or ethnic markets, and are widely used.

Their popularity has grown, and I have included several of the more familiar ones in this book as health enhancers.

Herbal medicine is a discipline in its own right, and remedies can be used for self-help and prevention. Self-diagnosis is not recommended for anything other than minor everyday ailments, and a professional medical diagnosis should be sought whenever there is doubt.

Herbs have powerful properties and they must be used wisely.

Herbs are easy to use for minor ailments, but serious problems need a consultation with a qualified medical herbalist who will refer the patient to an orthodox doctor if he or she thinks this is the best course of action.

There is a lot of confusion about the way drugs interact with herbs, and it is advisable to consult a medical herbalist if you are on medication. However, many mainstream doctors can't give advice on herbs or plant medicine because they do not study herbalism in medical school.

Both branches of medicine, scientific and traditional herbal medicine, can be used together, but a doctor also qualified in herbalism must be sought.

Natural healing has seen a renewal of interest in the West, and if you wish to learn about "green medicine" and how to use nature's healing herbs therapeutically, there are many good books on this subject.

You could also take a course on the topic, for educational purposes and for the enjoyment of learning about the fascinating world of herbs, plants and their beneficial uses.

The herbalist often has a quaint image as someone who gathers armfuls of plants and herbs from their garden or from fields, spending time boiling them up to make weird and wonderful concoctions.

The "herb wives" who gathered these plants and who made healing potions for the sick were persecuted by the physicians, priests and monks who took over herbal medicine and marginalized them.

Even today, herbal medicine is associated with spells and witches, and it is sometimes denigrated and mocked by many in the scientific community.

Thankfully, this image is slowly fading, as the use of herbs and plants for medical purposes is now becoming accepted as a usable form of healing. This is especially so for degenerative and chronic diseases that medical science has been unable to conquer.

While there are thousands of plant species in the world, very few have been investigated, but medical science has begun to show an interest in the active properties of plants. Many studies have been conducted that have confirmed the beneficial value of several herbs.

Plant-based medicines were the most prescribed treatments by doctors during the early years of the twentieth century.

With new scientific discoveries in chemistry and the growth of the pharmaceutical industry, however, very few of these plant-based medicines continue to be used.

Synthetic drugs became the first choice in the treatment of any disease. Science isolated the active ingredient of a plant and produced synthetic equivalents, and scientists argued that their drugs were safer, as they had undergone rigorous testing.

Herbalists claim that the whole plant should be used, as this means that all of the plant's properties work in co-operation and it is, therefore, a more natural way for the body to absorb the herb's curative qualities.

It is also believed that other parts of the plant provide checks and balances, providing safeguards and preventing side effects.

When a plant's single ingredient is isolated in a laboratory, it may become too powerful, or it may lose its potency.

This has happened with the plant ephedra. When the active ingredient was isolated, it was found to raise blood pressure, but herbalists had greater success when using the whole plant.

It seems that Mother Nature still has many secrets that she has not yet divulged.

There is a growing interest in an approach that aims to treat the whole person and not just the disease. This is called holistic medicine, where the mind, body and spirit are looked at in conjunction, and any imbalances are brought back into equilibrium.

Herbalists look to the cause of the problem rather than just treating the symptoms, seeing the mind, body and spirit as parts of one whole.

Herbalism and its beneficial curative properties are enjoying a revival today in the Western world as people look for gentler medicines that consider the whole person. There is no reason why "green medicine" and orthodox medicine cannot work together for the benefit of mankind.

CHAPTER 2

HOLISTIC HEALTH and HEALING

In the grave of a Neanderthal man in Iraq, grains of flower pollens were found thickly scattered in the soil surrounding this cave man's bones, indicating that these plant fragments may have been used for medicinal purposes.

There are no people in any part of the world who have not practised healing using plants, but recently, we have had to fight to retain the right to use herbs and plants for health purposes.

The philosophy of herbalism is:

"Prevention is better than cure."

The phytotherapeutic products used originate from plant roots, stems, flowers or leaves and they can take the form of liquid extracts, capsules, tablets or teas. They can also come from a herb garden, where the plants are grown on fertile, organic soil so that they are rich in nutrients.

Herbalists believe that plants have energy, and when grown in a healthy environment, their benefits are maximized. Some herbalists also plant and pick their herbs according to the cycles of the moon.

Anyone who has a garden can plant herbs and watch them grow, and can use them for culinary or medicinal purposes.

With growing awareness of the importance of respecting the earth's ecological balance, the wisdom of herbalism, its healing benefits and gentle therapeutics will no doubt continue to enjoy a revival.

Choosing the right herb or plant for the remedy is a skill that medical herbalists have acquired after years of study. This does not mean that herbalism is only for the qualified herbalist; anyone wishing to use these wonderful therapeutic plants can do so by either growing them in their garden or buying them from reputable companies.

Nature's pharmacy has a herb or plant for many conditions.

Some herbs function as nature's antibiotics, while others strengthen the immune system. There are those that help to improve mild ailments and yet others that can help boost energy or calm nervousness.

The exciting thing about herbs and plants is that they have many functions rather than just one, so a single herb may be used to prevent a cold and at the same time be used for a different problem.

I have chosen some popular herbal remedies that are easy to obtain or grow. Some of the more exotic ones are only available as supplements.

THERAPUTIC HERBAL BATHS

Herbal baths are used to enhance general wellbeing.

Herbal baths help to combat the pain of rheumatism or arthritis, alleviate eczema, psoriasis, colds and aching muscles.

Even if they are not used for a specific condition, they can enhance general health if taken regularly and specific healing herbs are used.

Water has long been believed to have curative properties, and when blended with herbs, the combination creates a powerhouse of healing.

Baths are easy home treatments that can be used to help combat many everyday ailments that cause pain and discomfort, despite not being severe health issues.

These baths and treatments soothe, vitalize and beautify. Herbs can be wrapped in a muslin bath bag and dropped into the bathwater.

Leave the herb bag in the bath while you are running the water. The wet bag can then be used as a wash flannel.

Some herbs, such as chamomile, can be made into a tea, and the solution can then be poured into the bathwater.

herbal BATHS for COLDS and FLU

Bathing in herb-infused water, with the addition of the appropriate healing herbs, is a therapeutic experience.

Warm, decongestant baths help cold and flu symptoms. Some of the best herbs to use for this purpose are those that help perspiration, thus speeding up metabolism.

Drink plenty of water to keep fluid levels up if you choose this kind of bath.

PEPPERMINT

Stimulating and a decongestant, peppermint helps to clear blocked nasal sinuses.

SAGE

The antiseptic properties of sage help eliminate muscular tension, relieve aches and pains, and ease congestion.

(Note: Do not use sage if pregnant.)

relaxing BATHS to help you SLEEP

When you feel tense, stressed and unable to sleep, let a relaxing hot bath steeped with lavender and chamomile relieve tension, calm nerves and bring restful feelings that will soothe your mind.

For a sleep-inducing bath just before bed, add some soporific herbs whose calming action and comforting vapours will relax you.

After a bath with these soothing herbals, you should be ready to enjoy a restful night.

LAVENDER

This herb has a settling effect on the nervous system, helping to calm anxiety and tension, leaving you feeling more peaceful.

CHAMOMILE

Use this herb when feeling restless, anxious or unable to relax.

A BLEND OF LAVENDER AND CHAMOMILE

This can be made in advance and added to the bathwater so that their blended properties can help you unwind as the ingredients get to work.

SITZ BATHS

The healing properties of herbs have also been used in sitz baths.

These special baths are used for pelvic, abdominal and back problems. For these purposes, a hip bath or tub is usually used.

The person sits upright with the water up to the waist. Used regularly in European spas and nature treatment centres, naturopathic doctors and herbal practitioners also use sitz baths for their patients.

There is nothing like the pleasure of submerging yourself into a warm, fragrant bath and enjoying a long soak when tension makes you feel low.

Herbs aid recovery in mind and body.

As you soak, the aromatic vapours released into the air and water can smooth and soothe the skin, deodorize the body, relax the nerves or stimulate flagging energy, depending on the herb you use.

HERB PILLOWS

Another interesting way to use herbs can be in herb pillows. Popular ones are usually made with lavender, due to its soothing, calming aroma.

If you have difficulty sleeping, as many people do in this frantic world, a lavender pillow is very tranquillizing and sleep-inducing.

CHAPTER 3

NATURAL ALTERNATIVES to ANTIBIOTICS

When antibiotics were discovered, it was thought that we would no longer be troubled by infections. The drugs developed in the 1940s were hailed as a panacea, and a whole range of antibiotics has been developed since then; they are now the most commonly prescribed drugs in the world.

Unfortunately, the efficacy of antibiotics has now lessened due to their over-use. This has resulted in bacteria fighting back in order to survive.

It was not envisaged that these smart little bacteria would evolve and develop resistance to most of the antibiotics we have today. Consequently, some infections require double the amount of antibiotics to combat them, and in some cases, even that is no longer effective.

This poses serious problems because diseases once thought of as extinct are re-emerging.

Today, mankind is suffering from a plague of super-bugs that are resistant to even the most potent antibiotics. Antibiotics are also ineffective in the treatment of viral infections.

Due to this severe threat to human health, medical science is beginning to look at plant medicines and to study antibiotics found in nature. A worried public is also looking to the plant world for effective bacterial and viral fighters. Nature's antibiotic properties are found in many herbs and plants.

Here are some of **Mother Nature's** star performers:

ANDROGRAPHIS

Used in Ayurvedic medicine for thousands of years, this herb has powerful antibacterial and antiviral properties. In Ayurveda, also called "The Science of Life", it is known as nature's antibiotic. Chinese healers have also used this valuable herb traditionally for respiratory infections.

Although andrographis was relatively unknown in the West, it is now appearing on the shelves of good health stores, and in the UK, even some GPs have begun to prescribe it in place of antibiotics.

ECHINACEA

Known as Indian snakeroot by Native Americans, this herb has become extremely popular as an antibacterial, antibiotic and antiviral. It is also one of the best herbal immune-system enhancers.

Taken at the first sign of a cold, it can alleviate the symptoms or even stop a cold from developing. Used to combat infections, it is a very useful herb to have in the home pharmacy.

GARLIC

A respected remedy the world over, garlic has been used medicinally for thousands of years.

It is a most effective antibacterial, antiviral plant. Used for bronchial and lung infections, colds, flu and sinusitis, its antibiotic properties
are well known.

OLIVE LEAF EXTRACT

Known as "The Tree of Life", olive leaf extract is a rich source of many beneficial compounds and potent antioxidants. The leaves have antibacterial and antiviral properties, and many cultures throughout the world have used this plant for nutritional and medicinal purposes.

Olive leaf is used to boost the immune system and is especially suitable for those who suffer from recurrent infections.

CHAPTER 4

HERBAL IMMUNITY

Plants are potent tools that help maintain health; they are very adaptable and can be used as foods and as medicine. In rhythm with the energies of the body, herbs are oriented towards health rather than disease. Healthy people take herbs to stay well.

This plant-based approach,
as we will see, is in tune with the immune system, the body's defender that helps to protect us daily.

Via this amazing system, the body protects itself against bacteria, viruses and other disease-producing micro-organisms.

It is vitally important that this system is kept in a state of balance. Too weak, and it will be unable to fight off dangerous infections; too strong, and it may fail to recognize the body and attack it, as in auto-immune disorders.

With the use of herbal protectors, we can keep the immune system functioning well.

In nature's pharmacy, some herbs function as protectors and immune boosters. To help the body stay in balance, these helpful herbs with therapeutic properties assist the immune system to continue with the vital work that it performs.

The following herbs are known to support the **immune system:**

ASTRAGALUS

This herb is used in Traditional Chinese Medicine as a tonic and an immune booster.

Due to its warming yang qualities, astragalus is an excellent herb to use during the winter season, when colds and flu germs abound.

Taken as a preventative for short periods, astragalus can keep the immune system working well.

ELDERBERRY

This rich, dark purple berry has been used for hundreds of years in Europe and has proven health-supporting properties.

Elderberry is full of flavonoids – a significant group of plant substances – and due to its antiviral action, is good to take during the winter season as a preventative, or if you feel you are succumbing to a cold or flu, to stop it in its tracks.

GOLDENSEAL

This is a broad-spectrum antibacterial and antiviral that has become very popular. Long before the advent of antibiotics, this herb was used to treat infections.

Today goldenseal is used to treat colds, flu and inflammation of the mucous membranes. It contains a powerful antimicrobial compound called berberine that is believed to have antibiotic action.

Effective against many infections, goldenseal is an excellent herb to use for maintenance of health during the winter. This herb is often coupled with echinacea to maximize its effect.

SIBERIAN GINSENG

The root of Siberian ginseng (*Eleutherococcus senticosus*) is highly revered as a herbal medicine, but do not confuse it with American ginseng (*Panax quinquefolius*).

Siberian ginseng has been used for thousands of years in Traditional Chinese Medicine as a "qi" energy (life force) herb.

It helps improve the immune response, enabling this system to fight off infections. It also acts as a general tonic, building strength and enhancing immunity, while its antiviral properties help to maintain overall health.

CHAPTER 5

HERBS that RETURN US to NORMALITY

Herbalists believe that many diseases are caused by an imbalance in the body, which may be due to several factors, such as stress, lack of exercise, faulty diet, lack of nutrients, lack of sleep or poor breathing. This is like the Traditional Chinese Medicine philosophy of the yin/yang balance, where a suitable herb will be prescribed to restore equilibrium.

The objective is not only to deal with the symptoms, but also to find the cause, and to help the patient work out a more satisfactory way of living that would build up the body's strength and natural resources.

This approach aims to strengthen and fortify the person and bring them back into a state of wholeness.

After taking down a detailed history, a qualified herbalist will work out a plan using the appropriate herbs according to the condition being addressed.

The patient is encouraged to be an active participant in his or her own health, rather than just a passive recipient of healthcare. Herbalists believe in this empowerment model.

Some herbs have a stimulating effect on the body, and others act in the opposite way. These herbs disperse stagnant energy, encouraging the repair of any damage and enhancing any functions that could work in a better fashion.

This concept is the total opposite of the analytical approach taken by Western medicine.

The following herbs fortify the **whole organism,** gently improving its function:

CINNAMON

This pungent herb with its sweet, aromatic smell is used in Southeast Asia to treat fever and flu.

Cinnamon has strengthening properties, is antimicrobial, anti-spasmodic, and it helps to protect against fungal infections.

The bark is used to create a warming, comforting drink. Crush a cinnamon stick and drop the crumbled herb into a teapot. The tea has a sweet, soothing taste. This herb helps to reduce infections in the respiratory tract, as it is naturally astringent and helps relieve nausea.

Those with pre-diabetes can use it to help regulate blood sugar.

MILK THISTLE

Milk thistle enhances overall liver function, promotes new cells in the liver, and it is known as a liver tonic.

Rich in a flavonoid called silymarin, research has found that this ingredient protects the liver, helping this important organ to combat damage from toxins, pollution, disease and alcohol abuse.

REISHI

An Oriental mushroom with a long history of traditional use, both in Chinese and Japanese cultures, it is also called "The Mushroom of Immortality".

Reishi has traditionally been thought to boost “qi” energy and is the most famous medicinal mushroom in the world.

It stimulates immune strength, supports liver regeneration, regulates blood sugar and enhances vitality. Believed to prolong a healthy life, reishi offers deep support to building up the body, strengthening and normalizing the system, especially after an illness.

ROMAN CHAMOMILE and GERMAN CHAMOMILE

These are the most widely used herbs and share nearly identical properties.

Both are relaxing, while Roman chamomile has a slightly more bitter taste and German chamomile has an analgesic action. These plants are strengtheners for the lungs, and their normalizing activities soothe nervous upsets.

The flowers can be used as a tea. Chamomile is brewed using the dried flowers, or you can use a teabag if you prefer. Add honey if the taste is too bitter. Teabags are available in health stores or specialist tea shops.

CHAPTER 6

ANCIENT ADAPTOGENS and TONICS

The term adaptogen was used by scientists to describe the active substances in plants that help bring about balance in the body systems.

These ancient herbal adaptogens and tonics are plants that have been used for thousands of years to nourish, repair and support the body's energies, helping it to return to a state of wholeness.

They are herbal regulator tonics that nature has provided for use as medicines.

Adaptogens and tonic herbs are used to help people stay well. They act slowly, enhancing overall health and wellbeing, and are taken to promote longevity.

Used as a preventative before developing an ailment, adaptogens can help inhibit many problems before they set in.

Adaptogens are known to strengthen the whole body and to return it to "normal". These herbs also help the body to counter the adverse effects of stress.

Not all stress is bad, but when people become fixed on a stressful situation, this can result in stress-related illness.

Many people develop high blood pressure due to their inability to manage stress.

The use of an adaptogen can help to lower blood pressure, but if the blood pressure is too low, the same herb may raise it.

In Traditional Chinese Medicine, stress is believed to deplete energy ("qi"), and adaptogenic or tonic herbs can restore it. Ayurvedic medicine uses adaptogens, believing in the same principle.

I have listed some of my favourites, so when you are feeling under a lot of stress and pressure, the protective power of these herbs may help you cope. They are remarkably effective in strengthening and calming overactive nerves and feelings of tiredness. Herbal medicines work slowly, but you will feel the benefits after two or three months.

ASHWAGANDHA

This is one of Ayurveda's tonic herbs that is believed to have rejuvenating, restorative and revitalizing properties.

Ayurvedic doctors prescribe this herbal energizer to people who have a weakened constitution.

The root is mainly used for its medicinal actions that are reputed to increase energy, vitality and vigour in elderly people.

The tea is traditionally made from the leaves of ashwagandha, and it is used to build up stamina, especially in the elderly.

Used therapeutically to increase energy in exhausted states, due to its balancing effects, this herb can also be used as a calming remedy for insomnia and stress.

Supplements can be found in all good health stores.

Ashwagandha is sold in capsules, tablets, powder or tincture form.

KOREAN (Panax) GINSENG

This mystic root of the East, called "The Root of Heaven", is a natural remedy that comes from a wild forest herb and has been used for thousands of years by ancient cultures.

Believed to be a general energizer, ginseng helps build up the body's vitality and is taken to maintain good health.

Ginseng is renowned for its extraordinary, energy-giving properties. Traditional Chinese Medicine believes that many varieties of ginseng are able to strengthen the body's vital energy ("qi"). These include Oriental red, white and American ginseng. Panax ginseng is the most popular.

Ginseng is one of the most useful adaptogens, as it contains many active compounds, vitamins, minerals and amino acids. TCM believes the long-term use of ginseng protects against degenerative diseases.

Although this herb is not specific to Ayurvedic medicine, it is one of the rejuvenating herbs used in India for its tonic actions, for low energy and for those who tend to feel the cold.

Taken as a tea made from the root, you would need to take ginseng for several weeks to benefit from its balancing and restorative powers. It is good to take in the autumn, and after a month or so, you will notice an improvement in energy levels that can be useful in the coming winter.

Use as a supplement or as a tea to help charge your energy points.

RHODIOLA ROSEA

Also known as Arctic or golden root, rhodiola rosea has been used in traditional European and Asian medicine systems for more than 3,000 years.

Rhodiola rosea helps to balance stress, stimulate the nervous system, eliminate fatigue, reduce mental fog and remedy lack of concentration. It is also believed to help mild depression.

This amazing botanical grows in the cold, mountainous regions of Europe and India. Its adaptogenic qualities are thought to help strengthen the immune system, and the roots have a unique ability to protect the body against stress, enabling it to adapt to demanding conditions and harmonize the body systems.

CHAPTER 7

ANTI-AGEING HERBS

For thousands of years, ancient cultures have used herbs for anti-ageing purposes. People dread getting older because it likely means a declining memory and the possibility of developing degenerative diseases.

The good news is that there are herbs in nature's pharmacy that can help to slow down the ageing process. Using nature's herbs helps us to grow older without growing old. The use of these natural marvels can allow us to remain in a state of youthful maturity for a long time.

In my opinion, using herbal medicine will go a long way in helping us stay healthy, look younger, remain active and retain an agile mind for many years.

GINKGO BILOBA

Rich in flavonoids and antioxidants, this ancient remedy helps keep the brain youthful by providing a better supply of oxygen and nutrients to this vital organ.

In this way, ginkgo appears to assist in preventing age-related memory loss, a common problem with advancing years.

The leaves and kernels have regenerative powers, and its antioxidant action protects against free radicals and oxidative stress.

GOTU KOLA

This herb, used in Ayurvedic medicine, is believed to have anti-ageing actions and strong energizing properties.

Rich in flavonoids, gotu kola has been used for thousands of years in India to extend lifespan and improve memory. It appears to support the connective tissues of the skin, increasing the integrity of the lower layers.

These inner layers provide the support structure of the skin, keeping it firm, strengthening the underlying network and preventing sagging. This herb appears to have a healing effect on these inner structures, nourishing the skin and enhancing collagen production.

EVENING PRIMROSE OIL

Native to North America, this plant and its root have long been used medicinally. Principally, we use the seed oil, which contains GLA (gamma-linolenic acid); this valuable ingredient is the special, essential fatty acid of the plant that is critically important to the body's functions.

Evening primrose oil (EPO) has become a most popular supplement with women, who use it medicinally for menstrual and menopausal problems. Taken for anti-ageing purposes, EPO is used for its age-defying effect on the skin. It supports the natural functions of this vital organ, minimizing premature wrinkling.

EPO can even repair the damage if this has already occurred; the prized oil from the seeds is rich in nutrients and contributes to the health of the skin, keeping it looking youthful and wrinkle-free.

AMLA

Also known as Indian gooseberry, this is an Ayurvedic herb used for anti-ageing purposes, due to its rich antioxidant content, which is believed to delay ageing and extend life. It is one of Ayurveda's main rejuvenating herbs.

Full of valuable nutrients, vitamin C, iron and calcium, amla can promote healthy skin by firming it and reducing premature signs of ageing.

It is one of nature's most potent revitalizing herbs, and it offers several beauty benefits for the skin as well as hair, improving its texture, strength and growth.

THE LEMON CURE

This is a true story about a friend of mine, and while it relates to a fruit rather than a herb, it just goes to show how useful ancient folklore can be, even in a dire situation. In this case, the legend came from Naples.

Laura and her husband were on a Mediterranean cruise that turned out to be the holiday from hell. Many people on the ship fell ill, including Laura, and within days, what had started out as holiday diarrhoea was starting to look more like dysentery. She was in a lot of pain, she was passing blood, and nothing that she had in her first-aid kit was helping.

Laura went to the ship's doctor, and the uninterested man flung her a pack of suppositories to use. Suppositories are rarely if ever used in the UK, but they are common in Europe.

The idea is that, as the medicine doesn't go through the stomach, it is supposedly easier for the body to deal with, and is therefore more likely to do some good if the patient is being sick.

However, Laura wasn't being sick, but she had severe diarrhoea, so while the idea of using the suppositories didn't appeal to her one bit, she also couldn't see how they would stay put long enough to do any good!

The Neapolitan valet who looked after the cabin came up with a workable solution. He brought Laura a glass of bottled spring water, to which the juice of half a really fresh lemon had been added, along with sweeteners to

make the drink palatable. He gave her a supply of lemons, water and sweetener and told her to make up this drink every two hours, and to keep on with the cure, taking the drink three or four times a day, even when she felt better. He told her that sugar would have made the situation worse, hence the sweeteners.

The lemon cure worked and, soon enough, Laura recovered enough to enjoy the second week of her holiday.

From that time on, if Laura or any member of her family suffers from tummy trouble on holiday, Laura immediately sets them up with **"The Lemon Cure"!**

CHAPTER 8

HERBAL GARDENS

If you have an outdoor garden, you can have fun growing any number of herbs. Even the smallest garden can include these fascinating plants.

Most herbs are quite hardy and do not need much looking after. If you do not have a garden, you can still grow herbs on a kitchen windowsill or in a window box. The wonderful thing about herbs is they are easy to grow either in an outdoor garden or in your kitchen, and they can be used for culinary purposes, or medicinally for many everyday ailments.

So, in your herbal medicine chest or in your kitchen larder, nature's herbs can be used for their therapeutic benefits or for their outstanding flavour when added to many different dishes. Either way, with healthy eating in mind, if used in recipes, their medicinal properties will be a healthful addition to every meal.

We all have to eat, and the easiest way of all to reap the benefits of herbs is to add them to your food every day. There is no clear boundary between herbs as food or as medicine, so both can be used to keep us well.

As a food, nutrients that are essential for health and to strengthen us medicinally, also improve energy and balance all our body systems.

I love the herbs that grow in my creative herb garden. I lavish lots of care and attention on them and enjoy watching them grow. They reward me by producing lots of lovely items that I use for many things.

I notice that my cats love them, too! Cats display innate wisdom and tend to go to the herbs that they like, chewing the leaves quite regularly!

Herbs are not only rewarding, but they are also useful, fragrant and beautiful.

I hope you will enjoy growing and tending herbs as much as I do.

The best time to start growing herbs is not too early in the spring, when the weather can be unpredictable, thus damaging delicate plants. Some herbs used in cooking, such as bay, basil, chives, oregano, mint, parsley, sage and thyme, also have medicinal value. When used for culinary purposes, their therapeutic qualities will still be of added benefit.

Many herbs can be made into **teas, tinctures, inhalations** and **ointments**.

When planting herbs,
water them regularly but do not over-water, and use suitable, nutrient-rich compost. When the herbs appear, keep them well trimmed.

They need a moderate amount of light, so choose a convenient location. Ideally, they should be grown in a relatively sunny, partly sheltered area with well-drained soil. If they are to be grown in a window box, make sure that they are placed where there is a lot of light.

You can be as creative, original and imaginative as you want.

If you are hesitant to start planting herbs in the garden, never having done this before, the easy way to start is with growing pre-potted herbs that can be bought from any garden centre, or even from supermarkets.

If you are busy, this saves a lot of time and energy.

If you only grow herbs in your kitchen, basil, thyme, parsley, rosemary or bay will provide you with a continual, all-year-round supply.

For medicinal or culinary purposes, the first choice would be a herb freshly picked. However, this is not always possible, so storing and drying herbs would be the second choice.

Picking herbs in the early morning after the dew has evaporated is the best time.

With rosemary and thyme, if the leaves are to be used, they should be picked when the herb is about to flower.

Besides enhancing the flavour of food, these are medicinally useful as well.

The easiest way to dry herbs is to find a warm, dry place out of the light. Spread them onto a large piece of paper, making sure air can circulate.

Tie them into bunches and hang them upside down in a dark, warm place, precisely as the medieval herbalists and wise women used to do.

INFUSIONS

Made in the same way you would make a pot of tea, infusions are suitable for flowers, leaves, aerial parts and fine roots, berries, seeds and barks.

- Use ½–1 teaspoon of dried or 1–2 teaspoons of fresh herb in 250ml (9fl oz) of boiling water.
- Pour the water over the herbs, cover with a lid and leave to infuse.
- Flowers should be infused for 3–4 minutes. Leaves and soft aerial parts should be infused for 5 minutes.
- Woody or other hard parts take a bit longer – say 5–15 minutes.

The longer the herbs are left to infuse, **the stronger** the taste, but you can add some honey to sweeten if you like.

DECOCTIONS

This standard preparation is suitable for any recipe that requires the roots, bark, seeds, berries or hard chips of a plant to be used. These require a longer extraction time to access their healing properties.

- Use about 40g (1oz) of dried herbs or 60g (2oz) of fresh herbs.
- Simmer them steadily in 1 litre (1qt) of water for about 30 minutes.
- Cover the chopped herbs so you do not lose any of the goodness.

Allow to **cool, strain** and enjoy the fragrance and flavour.

TINCTURES

These are alcohol-based preparations made using traditional methods, and in this way, the full spectrum of the plant's activity is retained.

This method is used for herbs that release their properties in alcohol rather than in water.

- Use 25g (scant 1oz) of dried or 50g (1½oz) of fresh herbs.
- Use 250ml (9fl oz) of your chosen alcohol, which can be vodka, brandy or wine.
- Add 150ml (5fl oz) of hot water, not boiling, to the alcohol.
- Place the chopped or bruised herbs in a jar and cover with the liquid.

Close the jar with a tight-fitting lid. Keep it in a cool, dark place and shake daily. After two to four weeks, strain and squeeze the herbs through a fine muslin or cloth. Now you have a herbal tincture, best taken in half to one glass of water before food.

The advantage of tinctures over water-based preparations is that the herb produces a medicine that stays potent for many years.

An echinacea tincture would be an excellent immune booster in wintertime, or a mixture made from valerian would be good to take for a relaxing night's sleep.

Other suitable herbs would be oregano, rosemary or thyme.

Tinctures' benefits are swiftly available, as they are dissolved in a solution. This allows a rapid uptake, as the liquid is quickly absorbed within the body. They are also easy to swallow and digest. Many good tinctures are sold in health stores, if you do not want to try to make one yourself.

Here is a list of the main herbs used **medicinally** and for **culinary** purposes:

BASIL

This strongly scented herb has analgesic, anti-depressant, antiseptic and soothing properties.

The leaves can be made into an infusion that herbalists use to treat colds. The leaves are also made into cough syrups mixed with honey.

CULINARY USES:

Sweet basil, with its delicious scent and flavour, is a versatile herb. It has an affinity with tomatoes, and the chopped leaves added at the end of cooking time give an excellent flavour to soups.

Used in many Italian dishes, it goes particularly well with pasta.

GINGER

This plant has been valued as a culinary and medicinal plant for thousands of years.

A warming herb, it is used to stimulate circulation and digestion. Ginger tea made from the root is suitable for winter chills and colds.

It is also good for settling the stomach and for nausea in pregnancy.

CULINARY USES:

Ginger root is peeled by cooks, grated, minced or chopped. It is used in chicken or fish dishes, added to salad dressings and is excellent when used in a sweet and sour sauce or stir-fries.

Fruit salads, cakes and crumbles taste delicious with the addition of freshly grated ginger.

OREGANO

This herb from the Mediterranean region is a wild form of marjoram. With its spicy aroma, oregano has powerful antiviral and antibacterial properties.

The herb can be used as a healing agent during infections and to help shorten colds and flu.

CULINARY USES:

Used in regional dishes of many countries, this pungent herb is an ingredient in a lot of Greek food, such as moussaka, but also in sauces, aubergine dishes and with lamb or pork.

It is a real favourite in Italian cooking, such as in bolognaise and other pasta and pizza dishes.

ROSEMARY

This woody herb grows well in an outside herb garden. Due to its stimulating and warming qualities, rosemary is used to help wound healing and as a scalp tonic.

When made into a tea, it is bracing and uplifting.

CULINARY USES:

Because of its warm, resinous scent, rosemary gives a savoury tang to roast beef, lamb, pork and chicken.

Use sparingly because of its strong, pungent flavour.

PARSLEY

This well-known herb is used by herbalists for gout and arthritic conditions due to its cleansing and diuretic properties.

Parsley tea is made from fresh or dried leaves and can be drunk after a meal to improve digestion. It is also said to clean the blood.

CULINARY USES:

Familiar as a garnish, this herb, whether fresh or dried, can be used in sauces, scrambled eggs, raw in salads, sandwiches, pasta and fish dishes.

THYME

This sweet-smelling herb grows well outside because it is hardy. Thyme is antiviral and can be used for respiratory problems, due to its expectorant and antiseptic properties.

It is a potent antimicrobial herb, too, with drying qualities. Thyme is an excellent herb to use for stomach chills and chest infections. You can make up therapeutic thyme from the fresh or dried herb, and it is also a good tea drink to have during the winter.

CULINARY USES:

The strong character of thyme is an essential ingredient to bouquet-garni, which is the classic French flavouring for stocks, stews, marinades, tasty sauces and hearty soups. Use chopped in fish, meat, poultry and all kinds of food with a delicate flavour.

It can also be combined with sage and breadcrumbs and some butter to make a stuffing for chicken or turkey.

CHAPTER 9

MEDICINAL HERBAL TEAS

And the leaf thereof for medicine.

Ezekiel 47:12

Another way to use herbs is in herbal teas, which are flavourful, refreshing and can positively contribute to good health.

They do not contain caffeine or other dangerous chemicals, and they make a valuable contribution to a healthy diet if taken regularly.

Ancient cultures have known for thousands of years that teas made from herbs have health-giving properties as well as being refreshing, calming, warming or just tasting nice.

On the **Greek island of Ikaria,** people drink a thick, black herbal tea made from herbs they grow themselves. It includes wild mint, spleenwort, purple sage and several other herbs, but the full formula is a closely guarded secret.

These people enjoy good health well into their later years, and many live to be over a hundred. They attribute this to the black herbal tea that they regularly drink.

It must be very efficacious, because it has been said that this is the island where people "forget to die"!

Herbal teas are enjoying a revival, and there are many in specialist tea shops or health stores today.

Even supermarkets stock a number of them. There is a tea for every occasion, with therapeutic effects reported by fans of herbal brews.

Having said this, it is better to make tea from the herbs growing in a herb garden, because these retain more of their healthful properties than commercial, pre-packed tea bags.

Herbal teas can be made by putting the dried herbs into a warmed pot and pouring boiling water over them. Leave them to brew for about 4 minutes, then strain into a cup.

If the taste is too strong, add some honey, a slice of fresh ginger, a cinnamon stick or even a slice of fresh lemon. Homemade herbal teas generally taste better than shop-bought tea bags, but these can also be used if preferred.

Herbs brewed into healing teas from roots, barks, twigs or stems will need a decoction to release the deeper essences of the herb, as these are hard or coarse substances, and just dropping them into boiling water will not work.

CHAMOMILE

Chamomile is one of our most well-known herbs.

A tea made from chamomile is excellent for nervous tension, digestive upsets, loss of appetite, heartburn, indigestion and for irritable bowel sufferers.

This tea is also beneficial when taken last thing at night for anyone who has been suffering from sleeplessness.

Chamomile tea is brewed by steeping dried flowers in freshly boiled water.

DANDELION

Used by herbalists as a blood and liver purifier, dandelion is believed to remove excess fluid from the body that has resulted from liver problems. It can be used as a digestive tea to increase the production of bile. Bitter-tasting herbs have long been used in herbal medicine to aid digestion, and the fresh young dandelion greens can also be added to salads.

To make a tea, pour freshly boiled water over the herb.

There is a superstition that claims, if you eat a dandelion, you will wet the bed. To add weight to this story, the French actually call this flower *pissenlit*, which literally translates as "wet the bed"! This is apparently due to the diuretic qualities of the plant.

GINGER

Ginger is a warming spice, with a long history of use in Traditional Chinese Medicine. Ginger relieves nausea and motion sickness, and it can help ease a sore throat. The medicinal properties reside in the root.

If you want to take advantage of ginger's beneficial properties, you need to brew a decoction by grating 40g (1oz) of fresh or dried ginger root. Simmer for 10 minutes in 600ml (1 pint) of water. Sweeten with honey.

This decoction will have an intense flavour with strong medicinal qualities. You can find ginger tea and teabags in natural food stores, but they are not as strongly flavoured.

NETTLE

Nettle is a plant everyone recognizes but usually thinks is just a weed; nevertheless, it has some interesting medicinal properties. It is a strengthening blood tonic, and it has been used by herbalists to support the liver, cleanse the blood and staunch bleeding. The tea has a richness that tones the entire system.

If you want to make nettle tea using some leaves from your herb garden, boil some water, then toss in a handful of nettle leaves.

Cover the pan, turn off the heat and allow the nettles to steep for an hour. This will strengthen the flavour. Strain and chill.

Nettles have diuretic properties, so they can help those who suffer from fluid retention.

PEPPERMINT

Prized for its menthol vapours, this tea is used to aid digestion, ease nausea and calm the stomach cramps often experienced by people who suffer from irritable bowel syndrome. Scientific research conducted in Tufts University, Massachusetts, found peppermint has antibacterial and antiviral properties as well as a robust antioxidant action.

To brew a flavourful cup of peppermint tea, use some dried herb dropped into freshly boiled water. Steep, strain and allow it to cool.

Peppermint is traditionally used to cleanse the body, and it can also be useful during winter for extra defence throughout the cold and flu season.

SAGE

Rich in antioxidants, sage is a valued herb in many anti-ageing regimes. If you have been growing sage in your herb garden and hanging bunches tied with a cord to dry from your kitchen ceiling, you will have plenty of dried sage on hand from which to make a healing tea.

Sage's analgesic action will calm down frazzled nerves, so if you have a tension headache, a cup of sage tea will help ease the pressure.

Sage tea is made the same way as peppermint tea (see page 183).

This herb can dry up mucus and reduce post-nasal drip, so it can also be helpful for those who suffer from seasonal allergies.

THYME

Thyme tea is a potent antimicrobial that can soothe coughs as well as fight colds and infections. Taken regularly, this tea restores the nervous system and enhances immunity. Make a tea from the dried herb dropped into boiled water, then strain.

If you don't feel adventurous enough to make a herb tea from these plants, there are many herbal teas on the shelves of supermarkets and health stores, although their medicinal properties will be weaker than the ones made from fresh or dried herbs.

CONCLUSION

If my cats have a health problem, they instinctively eat some grass, which makes them sick but gets rid of whatever is bothering them, and soon they start to feel better. They are also known to pick and chew a herb or two that they like! These smart felines instinctively understand that the plant world has herbs that help them when they feel off colour.

Ancient cultures did not have the benefit of scientific laboratories, but they knew which plants were therapeutic and which plants were not.

This knowledge was gained through intuition, trials and observation. Herbal medicine is a sacred art rather than a rational science, and herbalists and healers must have sensitivity, a well-developed sense of intuition, and a strong instinct as to which plant is best to use for whatever the body needs to stay well.

Relatively late in the day, scientists are recognizing the importance of instinct, but they still tend to downplay the herbalist's claim that it is the intricate makeup of a herb that accounts for its effectiveness. This is the reason that herbs are so difficult to prove scientifically. Each herb is different from every other herb, due to growing conditions, the cycles of

the moon, the state of the soil in which the plant was grown, and so forth. Every year, the makeup of the herb differs slightly, and this confuses viruses and bacteria.

Medical science hasn't been able to defeat all diseases, and now is the time to accept that the plant kingdom has a lot to offer, and we must not allow this hallowed knowledge to be lost to the public. There are thousands of people the world over who still wish to use this form of medicine. Recognizing the sacredness of plants and herbs is an experience that belongs in the realms of intuition allied to experience and logic.

I hope you enjoy dipping into this book and getting the most out of your herbs.

Marlene's disclaimer

Use herbs with caution, especially during pregnancy, or if you or others have any medical condition. A qualified herbalist or a doctor qualified in herbal medicine must be consulted for any serious medical condition. Herbs are natural, but they are also exceptionally powerful remedies.

“Using herbs in the healing process means taking part in an ecological cycle.”

Wendell Berry